BREATHE…MOVE…MEDITATE

A PRACTICAL GUIDE WITH SIMPLE DAILY TECHNIQUES TO BALANCE YOUR BODY, MIND AND SPIRIT.

CLAIRE DIAB

Cover Photography: Courtesy of Paloma Suau
Location: Half Moon Beach, Encinitas, California
Jewelry Designed by Karla Refoxo - TulkuJewels.com

Written by Claire Diab, 2007. Published by Living Life Productions.
Ninth Edition 2022

Edited by Claire E. Diab

Diab, Claire
Breathe, Move, Meditate:
Simple Daily Techniques to Balance your Body, Mind and Spirit.

ISBN: 978-0-692-41681-5

NAMASTE

I Honor the Place in you
In which the Entire Universe Dwells.
I Honor the Place in you, which is of Love, of Peace,
of Light, and of Truth.

When you are in that Place in You,
And I am in that Place in Me,
We are one.

As you Move Forward on Your Journey; May you be Blessed, May
you be at peace; May you have Love in your Heart, and May you have
Health, Wealth, and Wisdom.

I wish you lots of laughter and love.

Namaste,

Claire ✳

For more Information, visit AmericanYogaAcademy.com and ClaireDiab.com

CONTENTS

HOW TO BREATHE, MOVE, MEDITATE THE YOGA WAY

1. Hatha Yoga, the physical aspect of Yoga, is a system of self-development. Perform the poses mindfully.

2. Practice in a private place where you will not be disturbed. Fresh air or a well-ventilated room is a necessity.

3. Nourish your body with movement 20-30 minutes a day, 10-15 minutes in the morning and 10-15 minutes in the evening or late afternoon. If possible, practice at a consistent time each day.

4. Yoga is to be practiced mindfully, being aware of never straining. Allow the weight of the body to work for you.

5. Yoga poses should be approached gracefully and held easily with full deep belly breathing. Come out of poses as slowly as you went into it.

6. You will need a pad, mat, blanket or towel on which to sit or lie. The color should be soft and pleasing to your eyes.

7. Wear loose, comfortable clothing. Remove any jewelry and watches that may constrict your freedom of movement.

8. Wait at least 2 hours after eating a heavy meal before you practice movement and meditation.

9. Use essential oils rather than perfume or scented lotions.

PREPERATION AND TIPS

Create a sacred space

> Turn off your phone
>
> Place mat or towel down
>
> Dim lights and light a candle

Breathe in a relaxed manner

> Full deep belly breaths
>
> Breathe 4 to 6 breaths in each pose

Relax through the movements

> Tongue at Fire Point: place tip of tongue gently on ridge behind two front upper teeth.
>
> Unclench your teeth and relax your jaw
>
> Keep your shoulders relaxed back and down

Move easily and gently from one pose to the next

> Never force or strain
>
> Bring the corners of your mouth toward your ears

Enjoy the sequence!

BREATHING TECHNIQUES

Breathing is a science of enlivening the life-force throughout the body. It is practiced throughout the day, as it helps with physical and mental endurance, balance, and energy.

The Breath is the life-force that keeps us alive.

Belly Breathing

Belly Breathing is the basis of all breathing techniques

BENEFITS:

Relaxes the body and calms the mind. Revitalizes and rejuvenates the entire body. Strengthens the abdominal muscles, diaphragm, heart, and lungs. Improves digestion and elimination. Very soothing during menstruation. Can be practiced during exercise, relaxation, meditation, and throughout the day whenever calming and/or enlivening energy is needed.

1. Sitting with your spine straight, or lying down on your back, take a few deep breaths. Relax.

2. With a slow and steady breath through the nostrils, inhale into the three chambers of your lungs: abdominal (expanding the belly); thoracic (expanding the rib cage); and clavicles (expanding the upper chest and shoulders).

3. Slowly exhale, emptying the lungs. Gently squeeze the abdominal muscles at the end of the exhalation to squeeze out all of the excess air.

4. Continue breathing in this way for 5 to 10 minutes, focusing on the sensation of breathing.

Sounding Breath

BENEFITS:

Same as the Belly Breathing, just more pronounced. The mind relaxes with the sound of the breath, which calms the body and mind. Sounding breath is relaxing and energizing.

1. Sitting with your spine straight, or lying down on your back, take a few deep breaths. Allow your body to be relaxed.

2. With a slow and steady breath, breathe through the nostrils, gently contract the back of your throat (the glottis), creating a soft and audible hissing sound. The sound is like a gentle snore as if you were in a deep, relaxed sleep. To learn how to create this sound, practice whispering "haaa" with your mouth open on the exhalation and inhalation. Feel the sensation of the breath in the back of the throat. Then close your mouth and breathe in and out through the nostrils creating the sounding breath.

3. Lengthen the breath as much as possible and focus on the sound. Repeat for 5 to 10 minutes. As you advance in your breathing practice, repeat breathing technique for longer periods of time.

SPECIAL NOTES:

- You may wish to hold the breath briefly at the top of the inhalation and/or at the end of the exhalation.
- Create a circular breath by connecting the inhalation to the exhalation. Allow the breath to create one continuous flow, visualizing a circle of light moving up the back of the body as you inhale, and down the front of the body as you exhale.

CONTRAINDICATIONS:

There are no contraindications.

This is one of the most healing breathing techniques for everyone.

(NOTE: All breathing techniques are best done before eating.)

Rhythmic Breathing

BENEFITS:

Purifies the lungs, blood and cells of the body. Performing this breathing technique strengthens the heart and regulates heartbeat. Provides stamina and endurance while climbing stairs, running or performing any other vigorous exercise. You will create internal balance and harmony, regulating the natural rhythms within the body.

1. Sit comfortably and close your eyes. Place your hands on your lap.

2. Breathe in through the nostrils 2 breaths in & 2 breaths out.

3. Maintain a steady rhythm.

4. The breaths in and out are performed with power and strength.

5. This breathing technique can be incorporated while climbing stairs, running, walking or engaging in any other activity.

SPECIAL NOTES:

- Practice this rhythmic breathing technique going up and down stairs.
- In the morning, sit at the side of your bed or on a chair with feet on the floor andperform rhythmic breathing 2-5 minutes.
- Walk in the afternoon for 5-10 minutes (preferably outdoors) matching the breaths with each step.

CONTRAINDICATIONS:

Untreated high blood pressure, emphysema or other lung conditions.

Alternate Nostril Breathing

BENEFITS:

Balances the right and left hemispheres of the brain, bringing a sense of peace and clarity to the mind. Balances two of the main energy channels along the spine through which lots of energy flows. Relaxes and revitalizes the body and mind. Develops concentration and prepares one for meditation.

1. Bring the right index and middle fingers together. Place these fingers in-between your eyebrows.

2. Close your right nostril with your right thumb and inhale through the left nostril.

3. Hold the breath, closing off both nostrils (use ring and small finger to close off left nostril).

4. Raise the right thumb and exhale through the right nostril, keeping the left nostril closed.

5. Inhale through the right nostril.

6. Hold the breath, closing off both nostrils.

7. Bring the ring and small fingertips to the palm of your hand and exhale through the left nostril, keeping the right nostril closed.

   Steps 2 – 7 complete one cycle. Begin again inhaling through the left nostril. Repeat 3 - 9 times or what is comfortable for you.

SPECIAL NOTES:

- Alternate Nostril Breathing is performed with a smooth, steady, and subtle breath.
- Relax into the rhythm and flow of the breath, without forcing or straining.

- If your raised arm gets tired, support it by holding your elbow with the opposite hand.

- Listen to your body for the appropriate rhythm of inhaling, holding, and exhaling. The rhythm will be different for each individual and will vary slightly from day to day. The standard suggested ratio is 2:8:4 seconds, that is, you inhale for a count of 2, hold for a count of 8, and exhale for a count of 4. (As you become accustomed to this practice, you can increase the ratio to 4:16:8.)

- The suggested practice is 15 to 20 minutes daily. You may wish to start with five minutes a day and build your practice gradually over a period of time.

- Maintain your focus on the forehead with eyes gently closed throughout the practice, especially when holding the breath.

CONTRAINDICATIONS:

Holding the breath should be minimized or omitted for those with untreated high blood pressure, abdominal inflammation, lung conditions, or hernia.

Bellows Breath or Breath of Fire

BENEFITS:

Energizes, revitalizes, and recharges the entire nervous system by flooding it with a fresh supply of oxygen and energy. Brings mental clarity and alertness, massages the abdominal organs, and stimulates digestion and elimination. Strengthens the diaphragm, heart, and nerves. Removes toxins and stale air from the lungs.

1. Begin in a comfortable seated position with the spine straight. Take a few deep breaths and relax.

2. Allow your arms to accompany the breath by raising them overhead, fingertips extending upward, while you inhale through the nostrils.

3. Exhale through the nostrils as you swiftly bring the arms down, with the elbows bent and tucked into your sides, clenching your hands into fists.

4. Begin with a slow, deliberate rhythm, gradually picking up the pace as you synchronize inhalations and exhalations with the movement of your arms.

5. On your last inhalation, hold the breath in and extend your arms overhead with your fingers interlaced, index fingers pointing upwards. Hold the breath as long as possible.

6. When you release the breath, allow your arms to float down to your sides as you focus your awareness on the forehead with your eyes gently closed.

7. You can do the Bellows Breath without raising your arms. You may want to place your hands on your belly.

SPECIAL NOTES:

- Do a few Belly Breaths first, before Bellows Breath in preparation.
- Do one or two cycles of 20 or more expulsions.

- The exhalation and inhalation are no deeper than a sniffle.
- If you find that you are short of breath, or you feel dizzy, stop and rest.
- If you are having difficulty with the rhythm of breathing, place your hands on your abdomen and press your belly in during the exhalation.
- Be sure to keep your chest and rib cage lifted off the diaphragm. Relax your shoulders and facial muscles.

CONTRAINDICATIONS:

Menstruation, pregnancy, colitis, inflammation in the abdominal region, recent surgery, untreated high blood pressure, or other lung condition.

Breathe

Feelings come and go like the clouds in a windy sky.
Conscious breathing is my anchor.

Thich Nhat Hanh

MORNING / EVENING YOGA ROUTINE:

Invigorating / Restorative Yoga

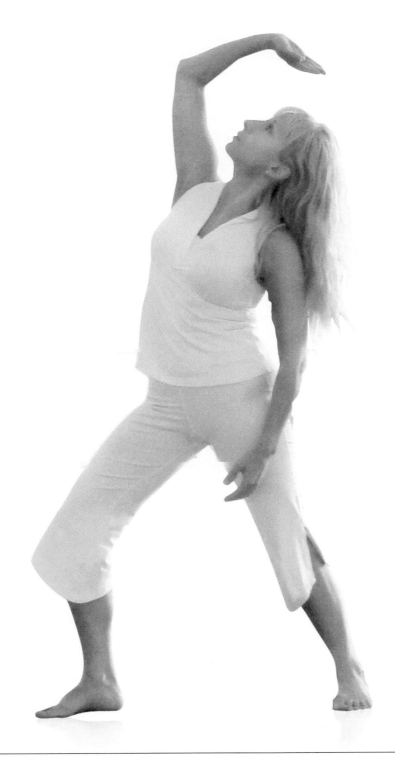

MORNING ROUTINE

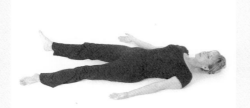

__1. LYING DOWN ON BACK__
Belly Breathing (15-20 times)

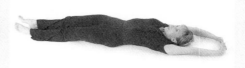

__2. FULL BODY EXTENSION__

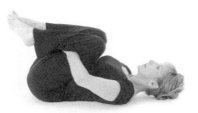

__3. KNEES TO CHEST__

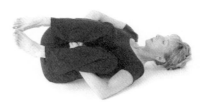

__3a. ROCKING RIGHT AND LEFT__
(6-8 times)

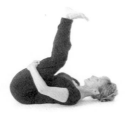

__4. FEET TO SKY POSE__
Flex Feet

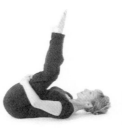

__4a. FEET TO SKY POSE__
Point Toes (6-8 times)

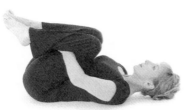

__5. KNEES TO CHEST__

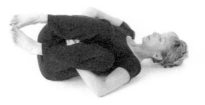

__5a. ROCKING RIGHT AND LEFT__
(6-8 Times)

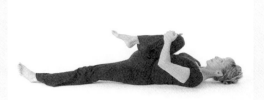

6. KNEE TO CHEST
Right Side

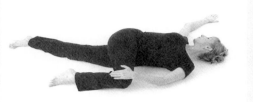

6a. KNEE DOWN TWIST
Right Side

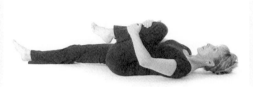

6b. KNEE TO CHEST
Left Side

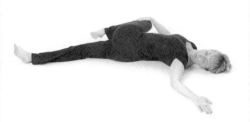

6c. KNEE DOWN TWIST
Left Side

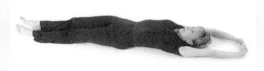

7. FULL BODY EXTENSION

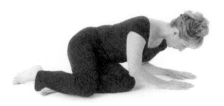

8. Sit Up (Transition)

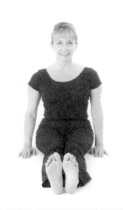

9. SEATED FORWARD

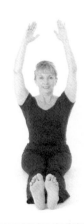

9a. INHALE: Arms Up

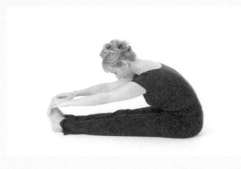

__9b. EXHALE: Hands Toward Toes__
(3-4 Breaths)

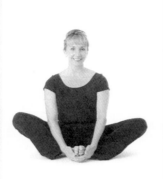

__10. BUTTERFLY__

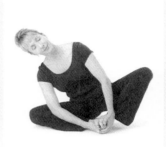

__11. ROCKING BUTTERFLY__
Rock Right

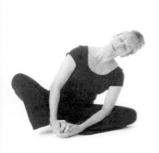

__11a. ROCKING BUTTERFLY__
Rock Left
(6-8 Times)

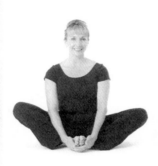

__11b. BUTTERFLY__

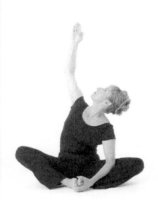

__12. REACHING BUTTERFLY__
Right Arm Up

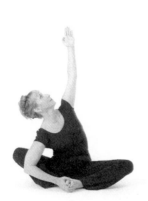

__12a. Left Arm Up__
(6-8 Times)

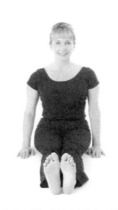

__13. SEATED TWIST__

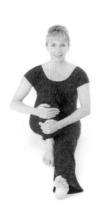

__13a. Right Knee In__

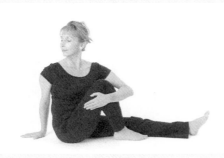

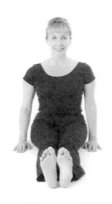

[Repeat 13a,b, c with Left Leg]

13b. TURN RIGHT
Left Arm Around Right Leg
Chin Over Right Shoulder

13c. SEATED FORWARD

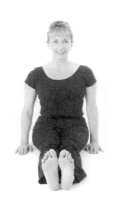

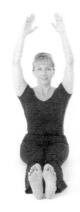

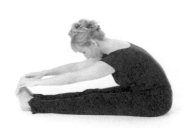

14.b. EXHALE: Reach Toward Toes

14. SEATED FORWARD BEND

14a. INHALE: Arms Up

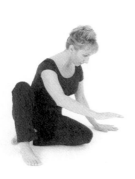

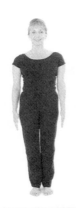

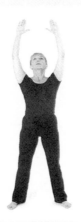

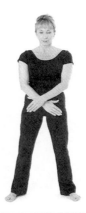

15. Stand Up
(Transition)

16. STANDING MOUNTAIN POSE

16a. INHALE: Arms Up

16b. EXHALE: Arms Down (4-6 Times)

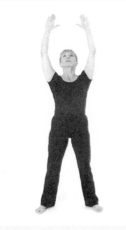

17. STANDING SUN
INHALE: Arms Up

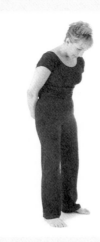

17a. EXHALE: Clasp Hands
Behind Back

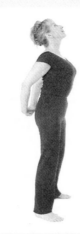

17b. INHALE: Bring
Arms Back
(4-6 Times)

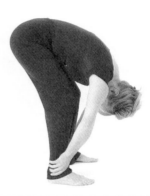

18. STANDING FORWARD
BEND

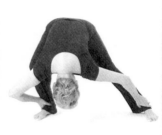

18a. SWAY RIGHT
Bend Right Knee

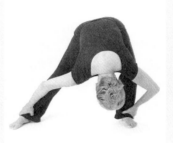

18b. SWAY LEFT
Bend Left Knee

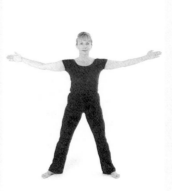

19a. FIVE-POINTED
STAR

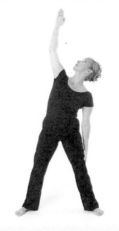

20. HALF TRIANGLE
Right Side

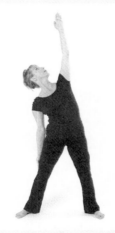

20a. HALF TRIANGLE
Left Side (2-4 Times)

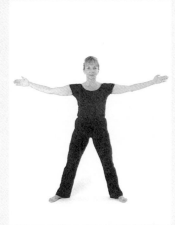

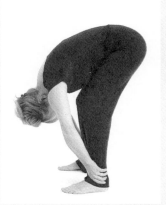

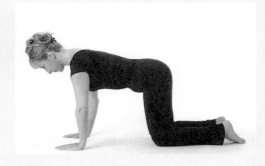

21. FIVE POINTED STAR

22 . STANDING FORWARD BEND

23. TABLE POSE
(Transition)

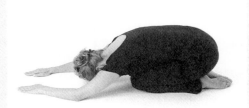

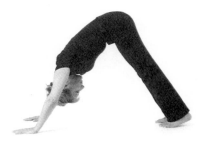

24. CHILD'S POSE

25. DOWNWARD DOG

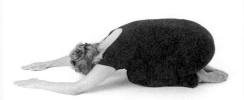

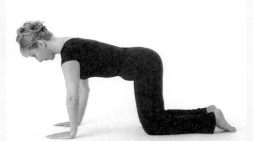

26. CHILD'S POSE

27. TABLE POSE

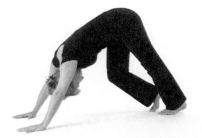

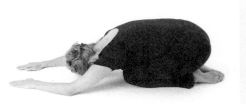

28. DOWNWARD DOG
Alternate Heel Raises
(6-8 Times)

29. CHILD'S POSE

EVENING ROUTINE

EVENING ROUTINE:

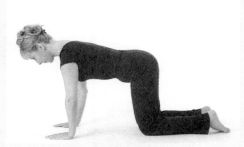

1. TABLE POSE

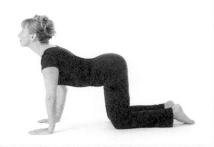

2. DOG POSE INHALE

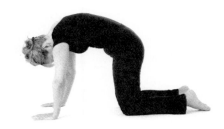

2a. CAT POSE EXHALE
[REPEAT DOG / CAT 8-12 TIMES]

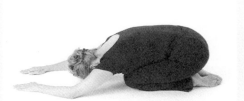

3. CHILD'S POSE

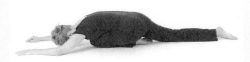

4. EARTH POSE
Right Leg Back

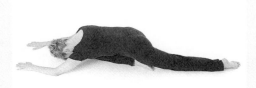

4a. EARTH POSE
Left Leg Back

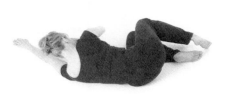

5. ROLL ONTO BACK Gracefully
(Transition)

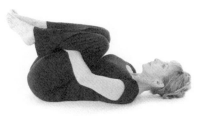

6. KNEES TO CHEST

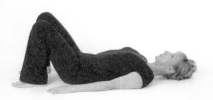

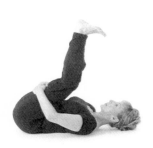 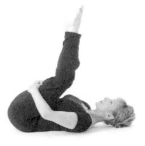

8. MOUNTAIN RAISES
FROM THE SEA

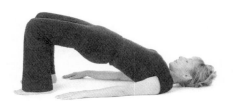

7. FEET TO SKY POSE
Flex Feet

7a. FEET TO SKY POSE
Point Toes (6-8 Times)

8a. EXHALE: Raise Hips
(4-8 Times)

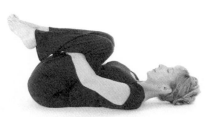

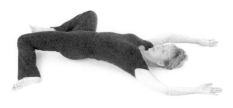

9. KNEES TO CHEST
Rock Right and Left

10. LYING DOWN HIP ROCKS
Right Side

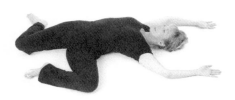

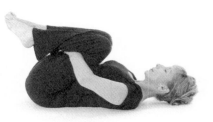

10a. LYING DOWN HIP ROCKS
Left Side

11. KNEES TO CHEST

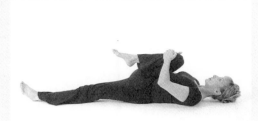

12. KNEE TO CHEST
Right Knee Toward Chest

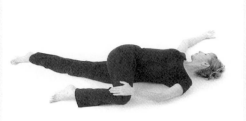

12a. KNEE DOWN TWIST
Right Knee to Left Side
Right Ear Toward Floor
(Relax Jaw)

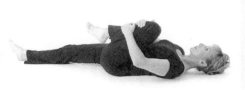

12b. KNEE TO CHEST
Left Knee Toward Chest

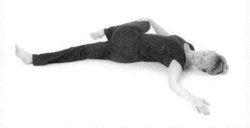

12c. KNEE DOWN TWIST
Left Knee to Right Side
Left Ear Toward Floor
(Relax Jaw)

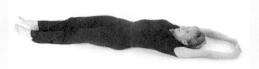

13. FULL BODY EXTENSION

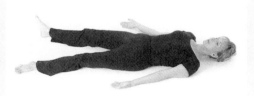

14. RELAXATION POSE

SUN SALUTATIONS I, II & III

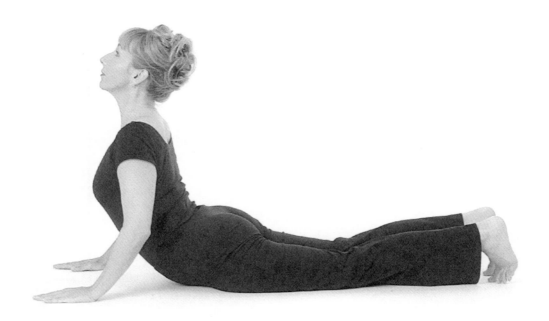

"Even after all this time,
The Sun never says to the Earth ...You Owe Me....
Look at what a Love like that does,
It Lights up the Whole Sky."

–Hafiz

Sun Salutations

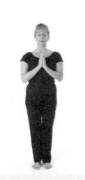

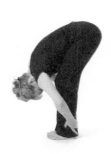

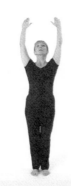

1. HANDS TO HEART POSE
Take a Few Deep Breaths

2. HANDS TO SKY POSE
INHALE

3. HAND TO FOOT POSE
EXHALE

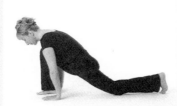

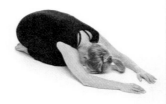

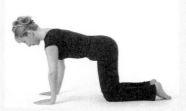

4. EQUESTRIAN POSE
INHALE
Left Leg Back

5. CHILD'S POSE
EXHALE

6. TABLE POSE
INHALE

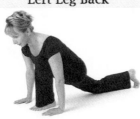

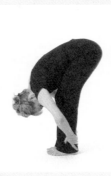

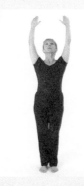

7. EQUESTRIAN POSE
continue to INHALE
Left Leg Forward

8. HAND TO FOOT POSE
EXHALE

9. HANDS TO SKY POSE
INHALE

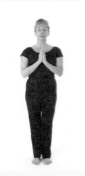

[REPEAT SERIES 6-8 TIMES, ALTERNATING SIDES]

10. HANDS TO HEART POSE
EXHALE

Sun Salutations

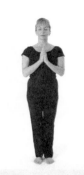

1. HANDS TO HEART POSE
Take a Few Deep Breaths

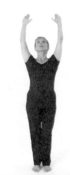

2. HANDS TO SKY POSE
INHALE

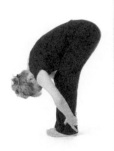

3. HAND TO FOOT POSE
EXHALE

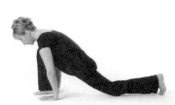

4. EQUESTRIAN POSE
INHALE
Left Leg Back

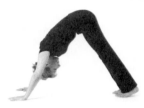

5. DOWNWARD DOG
EXHALE

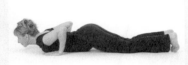

6. EIGHT LIMBS / PLANK
INHALE

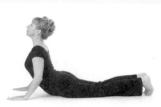

7. COBRA POSE
continue to INHALE

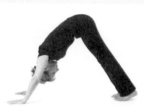

8. DOWNWARD DOG
EXHALE

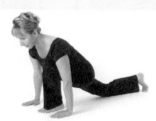

9. EQUESTRIAN POSE
INHALE
Left Leg Forward

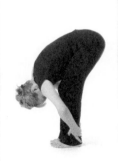

10. HAND TO FOOT POSE
EXHALE

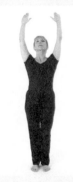

11. HAND TO SKY POSE
INHALE

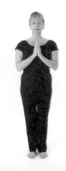

12. HANDS TO HEART POSE
EXHALE

Sun Salutations III with Mantras

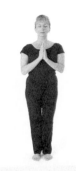

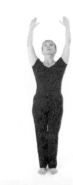

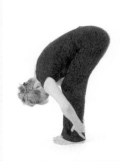

1. OM MITRAYA NAMAHA
(Om Mit-tri-yah Namah-hah)

2. OM RAVAYE NAMAHA
(Om Rah-vay-ya Namah-hah)

3. OM SURYAYA NAHMAHA
(Om Sir-yah-yah Namah-hah)

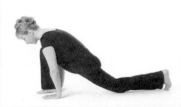

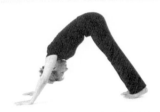

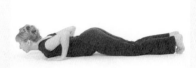

4. OM BHANAVE NAMAHA
(Om Bon-ah-vay Namah-hah)

5. OM KHAGAYA NAMAHA
(Om Kug-ah-yah Namah-hah)

6. OM POOSHNE NAMAHA
(Om Push-nay Namah-hah)

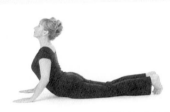

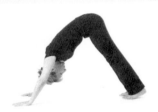

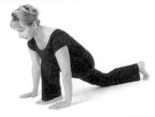

7. OM HIRANYA GARBHYA NAMAHA
(Om Her-ron-yah Gar-bah-yah
Namah-Hah)

8. OM MARICHAYA NAMAHA
(Om Mar-ree-chee-yah Namah-hah)

9. OM ADITYA NAMAHA
(Om Ah-dee-tee-yah Namah-hah)

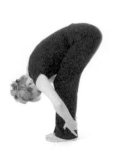

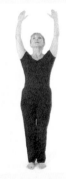

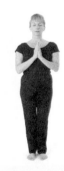

10. OM SAVITRE NAMAHA
(Om Sah-vee-tray Namah-hah)

11. OM ARKAYA NAMAHA
(Om Ahr-kay-yah Namah-hah)

12. OM BASKARAYA NAMAHA
(Om Buhs-kurah-yah Namah-hah)

CHAIR YOGA:

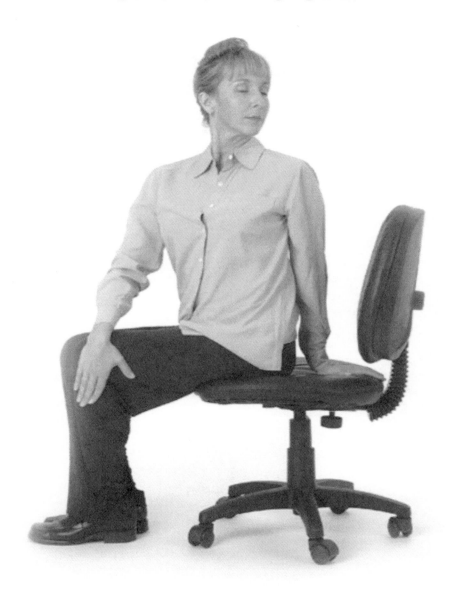

"To accomplish great things…
We must not only act… we must also dream…
Not only plan… we must also believe"

– Anatole France

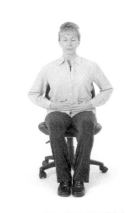

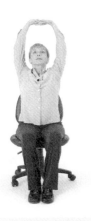

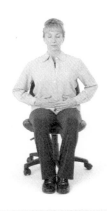

__1. COMPLETE BREATH__
(6-8 Breaths)

__2. ARMS UP__
Inhale

__3. ARMS DOWN__
Exhale
(Repeat 2 & 3 Two to Six Times)

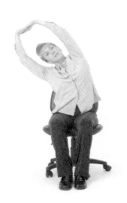

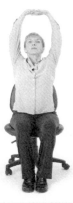

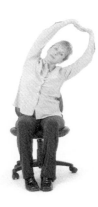

__4. SIDE BEND RIGHT__
Exhale

__5. CENTER__
Inhale

__6. SIDE BEND LEFT__
Exhale
(Repeat 4, 5 & 6 - Three to Six Times)

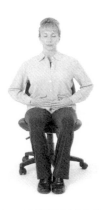

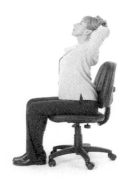

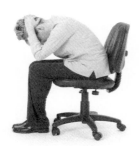

__7. REST__

__8. BACKBEND__
Clasp Hands Behind Head
Inhale

__9. FORWARD BEND__
Exhale
(Repeat 8 & 9 Three to Six Times)

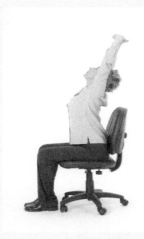

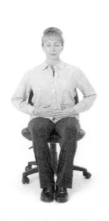

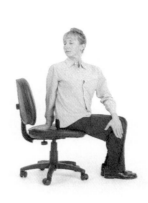

10. ARMS UP
Inhale

11. REST

12. TURN RIGHT
(Complete Breath 3-6 Times)

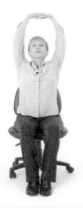

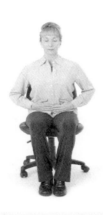

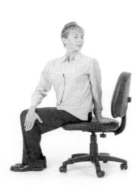

13. ARMS UP
Inhale

14. REST

15. TURN LEFT
(Complete Breath 3-6 Times)

[Repeat 10, 11, 12, 13, 14 & 15]

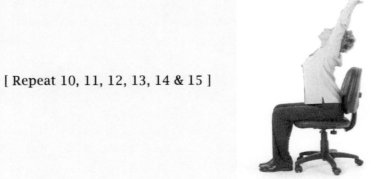

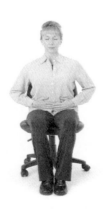

16. ARMS UP
Inhale

17. RELAXATION
3-5 Minutes

SIX DIRECTIONS OF THE SPINE

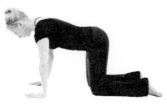

TABLE POSE

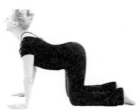

1. BACKBEND
Dog Pose - Inhale

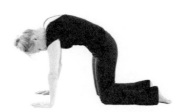

2. FORWARD BEND
Cat Pose - Exhale

[Repeat Backbend / Forward Bend 4-6 Times]

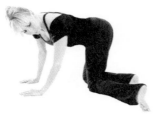

3. SIDE BEND RIGHT
Exhale

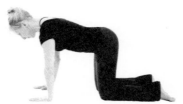

TABLE POSE
Inhale

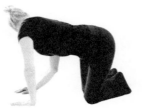

4. SIDE BEND LEFT
Exhale

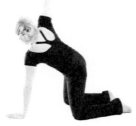

5. RIGHT ARM UP
TURNING RIGHT
Inhale

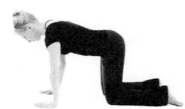

TABLE POSE
Exhale

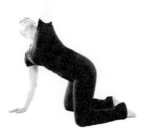

6. LEFT ARM UP
TURNING LEFT
Inhale

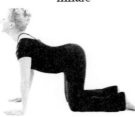

1. BACKBEND
Dog Pose - Inhale

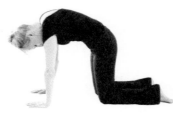

2. FORWARD BEND
Cat Pose - Exhale

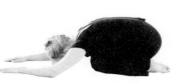

CHILD'S POSE
Rest

[Repeat Backbend / Forward Bend 4-6 Times]

MEDITATION

Meditation is the state of consciousness characterized by stillness and inner calm. When you change your inner world, your outer world will change.

I. BENEFITS OF MEDITATION

1. Experience peace of mind
    (the average person has over 50,000 thoughts per day). → *70-80% plus are the same thought leftover from yesterday*

2. Improves concentration and improves focus
    (you will be more efficient in the things you do).

3. Increases clear, positive thinking (see the glass as half full instead of half empty).
    ↳ stop being so negative

4. Increases intuition.

5. Increases energy.

6. Reduces stress levels.

7. Reduces aging process (catabolic and anabolic processes).

8. Experience present-moment awareness.

9. Experience a connection with Nature's Intelligence.

10. Develop ability to manifest intentions and desires.

11. Discover inner resources of power and knowledge.

12. Discover your true self.

II. HOW TO MEDITATE

1. Pick a time of day or evening that fits your schedule (AM and PM). Schedule an appointment with yourself.

2. Find and create a sacred place. Turn this space into a sanctuary.

3. Silence phone, cell phone, smart watches, computer, TV, etc.

4. Inform your family and friends that you will be meditating.

5. Sit comfortably with an upright spine (feet on ground or ankles crossed).

6. Have a clock, watch or set alarm on cell phone so you can keep track of time.

7. Softly close your eyes and say to yourself, "I will now meditate for___minutes."

8. Focus on the area of the mid-forehead or heart center.

9. Begin repeating your mantra easily and effortlessly.

10. If your mind wanders, gently and effortlessly come back to the mantra.

11. After your time is up, relax for a moment to settle into the stillness and silence before opening your eyes and moving back to activity.

30 - 60 seconds

III. WHAT MAY OCCUR WHILE MEDITATING

1. Your mind may become restless and active.

2. You may fall asleep.

3. You may experience stillness and silence.

"Meditation is the perfect way to purify and quiet the mind, which then rejuvenates your Body, Mind and Spirit."   – Claire Diab

	mon.	tues	wed	thurs	fri	S A T	sun
am	6:15 or 6:30	6:15 or 6:30	~~2~~ 2-2:15	6:15 or 6:30	8	10	10
Pm	9:30	10	10	11	11	11	9:30

CHI KUNG HEALING SOUNDS

Chi Kung (also spelled Qi Gong) is an ancient healing practice from China dating back 5000 years. It is the Art and Science of using Breathing Techniques, Gentle Movements, and Meditation to Cleanse, Strengthen, and Circulate the Life Energy "Chi" in and around the body.

Chi Kung is a powerful, practical tool that people can easily learn to relieve stress and tension and replace them with energy and vibrant health. It can also help get us back in touch with ourselves and our beautiful bodies, minds, and spirits. It enables us to break the negative habits we have acquired and replace them with positive ones that support our health and well-being. Chi Kung is a natural, easy form of self-care, which can make a difference in your life and how you feel everyday.

Each organ is surrounded by a sac or membrane called Fascia. The Fascia releases excess heat through the skin and brings in cool life-force and energy from nature. An overload of emotional or physical stress causes the fascia to stick to the organ, which then is not able to release its heat or toxins. The organs and skin can become clogged with toxins and the organs can become overloaded. These healing sounds release the heat and toxins.

CHI KUNG HEALING SOUNDS

Practice each sound 3 times, once a day. Practice on an empty stomach and allow yourself to rest for 3 to 5 minutes once you have finished.

DENSE ORGANS	HOLLOW ORGANS	SOUND
Heart	Small Intestine	Haaaaa
Lungs	Large Intestine	Ssssssss
Liver	Gall Bladder	Shhhhh
Spleen	Stomach, Pancreas	Whooo
Kidneys	Gall Bladder	Woooo
Triple Heater	Governing & Conception Vessel	Heeeee

NOTES

_____

_____

_____

_____

_____

_____

CHAKRA AWAKENING TECHNIQUE

Chakra is a Sanskrit word meaning "wheel of energy" or energy centers. We have **seven** main energy centers that run along the spine, starting at the base of the spine all the way up to the top of the head.

Chakras are junction points between our consciousness and our physiology. At each chakra, there are bundles of nerve endings which connect with our glands and organs. With attention, color, and vibration we create space around each chakra allowing the energy to flow more freely and effortlessly around each location and throughout the body.

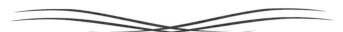

Let's begin at the **Root Chakra**. With your eyes softly closed, bring your awareness down to the base of your spine. Where your attention goes, energy flows. The nerve endings here go down through the legs. When there is space around this chakra we feel a sense of being more grounded, more stable and more connected to the earth. Each chakra is associated with a color. The beautiful colors of the spectrum which are all around us. The colors of **Red, Orange, Yellow, Green, Blue, Indigo, Violet**. We see them in a rainbow or when we hang a crystal in a window. The Root Chakra is associated with the color **Red**. Think, imagine, or feel a beautiful red illuminating the area of the root chakra. The healing vibrational sound for the Root Chakra is "Lam."

Breathe in…Exhale **Lammm**

The **Creativity Chakra**, located above the root and below the navel awakens us to our masculine and feminine energy which resides in all of us. The nerve endings here connect with our reproductive organs. When we create space here we feel the vibrancy and vitality which come from our creative sexual energy center. Keeping your eyes softly closed, breathing in and out, bring your awareness to the creative, sexual energy center. Think, imagine, or feel the beautiful color of **Orange** – Imagine breathing in the color **Orange**. The sound for the Creativity Chakra is **Vam**.

Breathe in… Exhale **Vammm**

The **Solar Plexus Chakra**, above the navel, below the heart, is your power energy center. Where we get our inner strength and power from. When there is space here, your inner strength and power will flow to you more easily and effortlessly. Think, imagine, or feel the beautiful color of **Yellow**, yellow golden light like the sun, solar power - breathe in the color **Yellow**. The sound for the Solar Plexus Chakra is **Ram**.

Breathe in… Exhale Rammm

The **Heart Chakra**, at the center of the chest, is where love and compassion flows to us and from us. When there is space here, love and compassion will flow more easily and effortlessly to you and from you. Think, imagine, or feel a beautiful **Green**, like an emerald or a forest, illuminating the area of your heart center - breathe in the color **Green**. The sound for the Heart Chakra is **Yum**.

Breathe in… Exhale Yummm

The **Expression Chakra**, the chakra in the area around your neck and throat, is responsible for expression and communication. When energy is flowing more freely around this chakra, we are able to express more easily and effortlessly who we are and what we want. Think, imagine, or feel a beautiful **Blue** like the sky or the ocean. The sound for the Expression Chakra **Hum**.

Breathe in… Exhale Hummm

The **Intuition Chakra**, the chakra in the area around your brain is where knowledge, wisdom, and insights come from. When energy is flowing more freely in and around your brain, knowledge, wisdom and insights will come more easily and effortlessly. Think, imagine, or feel a beautiful **Indigo** color, a dark blue, bluish gray purple. The sound for the Intuition Chakra is **Sham**.

Breathe in… Exhale Shammm

The **Crown Chakra**, the chakra at the top of your head, is where we connect with our beautiful spiritual essence which sparkles and shines through our eyes. When awakened your eyes will sparkle and shine more brightly now and forever more. It is here we feel the sense of oneness…where the sense of **I** becomes **We** and the sense of **We** becomes **Us** and we feel the oneness… the union… the yoga… within us and all around us. Think, imagine, or feel a beautiful **Violet** color illuminating the area around the top of your head. The sound for the Crown Chakra is the beautiful healing vibration of **Om** that connects us all.

Breathe in… Exhale **Ommm**

Breathing in, breathing out. Feel this beautiful, calm, peaceful, yet vibrant feeling within. Gently begin to move your toes and your fingers. If you are lying down, come up to a seated position.

Bringing your palms together, hands to heart pose. With your eyes softly closed, let's celebrate together with **Om**.

Breathe in… Exhale **Ommm**

Bringing your fingertips toward your forehead, bowing and acknowledging your beautiful body, your beautiful mind, and your beautiful spirit. Lifting back up bring your hands to your heart center. I wish you peace and happiness.

Namaste: I honor the light in you that is the same in me.

Namaste

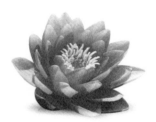

THE SEVEN SPIRITUAL LAWS OF SUCCESS

The Seven Spiritual Laws of Success by Dr. Deepak Chopra teaches us ancient Principles that we can use on and off the Yoga mat. Living these Principles will lead you to a life of true success and a deeper understanding of life and the Universe around us – a life of beautiful evolution, spiritual growth, and transformation.

The Seven Spiritual Laws of Success has changed my life in the most positive and beautiful way… this book has shaped how I look, how I feel, and how I live my life.

As we use these Principles in every aspect of our work, home, and in our relationships, we learn how to interact harmoniously and flow together beautifully. I am pleased to share the gifts in this book with you.

The Seven Spiritual Laws of Success

Day of the Week		*Principle of the Day*
1. Sunday	–	The Law of Pure Potentiality
2. Monday	–	The Law of Giving and Receiving
3. Tuesday	–	The Law of Karma or Cause and Effect
4. Wednesday	–	The Law of Least Effort
5. Thursday	–	The Law of Intention and Desire
6. Friday	–	The Law of Detachment
7. Saturday	–	The Law of Dharma or Purpose in Life

1. Sunday – The Law of Pure Potentiality

The Law of Pure Potentiality gives us a deeper understanding of our Spiritual Essence. We practice the Law of Pure Potentiality by quieting the mind and being present through meditation and taking time to be silent for a period of time each day. This Principle gives us a deeper connection with Spirit when we let go of judgements of people, places, and/or things – including ourselves. Spending time in nature also awakens us to our Spiritual Essence. Connecting with Nature's Intelligence awakens us to the Divine presence that is everywhere, and which shines through our eyes. Take time to be silent and just BE. Cultivate silence, spend time in nature, and witness the intelligence within every living thing, practice non-judgement.

1) Meditate 2 times per day (10-15 minutes).   2) Spend time in Nature.

3) Practice non-judgement.

MANTRA:
Om Bhavam Namaha   "I am Spirit."
[Om Bah-vam Na-ma-ha]

2. Monday – The Law of Giving and Receiving

The Law of Giving and Receiving helps us to keep energy flowing freely and keep abundance, affluence, and all good things flowing to us. A great example of Giving and Receiving is witnessing the breath moving in and out of the body. If you hold your breath in, you will notice how it becomes slightly uncomfortable. Even holding the breath out without inhaling becomes slightly uncomfortable too. If you stop the flow of either Giving or Receiving, you interfere with the natural flow of life. Today, bring everyone you meet a gift, a compliment, a smile. Meet the eyes of everyone you come into contact with, silently wish them love, joy, and laughter. Gratefully receive and acknowledge all gifts given to you, material or otherwise. Keep wealth and love circulating in your life by setting an intention to give and receive; there are gifts all around us, so be present and notice.

1) Give to everyone you encounter. 2) Receive all the Gifts life has to offer you.

3) Give the most precious Gifts of Love, Caring, Affection, Appreciation and Time.

MANTRA:
Om Vardhanam Namaha   "I am the nourisher of the Universe
[Om Var-dah-nam Na-ma-ha]   and the Universe nourishes me."

3. Tuesday – The Law of Karma or Cause and Effect

The Law of Karma says that out of infinity choices there is one perfect choice that will create happiness for yourself and all of those around you. Your body acts as an antenna which will send you feelings of comfort or discomfort. When presented with a choice or decision, ask yourself: "Will this choice nourish me?" Be present, notice your body's reaction, and listen. When you notice and acknowledge all of your choices, it becomes easy for you to make mindful decisions. Learn to choose actions that bring happiness and success to others, which will then, in turn, bring happiness and success back to you.

1) Ask yourself: "Will this choice nourish me?" 2) "How will this choice affect me?" 3) "How will this choice effect those around me?"

MANTRA:
Om Kriyam Namaha "My actions are aligned with the Universe."
[Om Kree-yam Na-ma-ha]

4. Wednesday – The Law of Least Effort

The Law of Least Effort can be thought of as The Principle of Allowing. When we have total acceptance of the moment, we manifest a creative response. Release the need to struggle against the whole Universe by struggling against the moment. In each situation, good or bad, there is a seed of opportunity. It is important to see and accept this. Losing a wallet may lead us into a different route than we had planned, or it may offer a lesson in being present and organized. The Principle of Least Effort allows us to accept our current situation as it is so we will have more energy for things that are important and worthwhile.

1) Practice acceptance. 2) Take responsibility. 3) Be open to all points of view.

MANTRA:
Om Daksham Namaha "My actions achieve maximum benefit
[Om Dahk-sham Na-ma-ha] with minimal effort."

5. Thursday – The Law of Intention and Desire

The Law of Intention and Desire brings us to the awareness that we are here to manifest our deepest dreams and desires. Everything we want, we already have… we simply must be open to the guidance received in the situations of our daily life.

Create a list of all the things you want to manifest; I keep mine in my wallet and look at it every day. My list begins with the desires I have for myself: physically, mentally, emotionally, spiritually, and materially. At the top of all my lists are "I am Strong," "I am Healthy," "I am Happy." What you think, you create, and what you think, you become. You can have all that you desire. Enjoy the journey of manifestation; the whole Universe is supporting you. Be clear of your intentions and trust the outcome, practice present moment awareness.

1) Make a list of your Intentions and Desires. 2) Read your list after meditating.
3) Practice present moment awareness.

> **MANTRA:**
> Om Ritam Namaha   "My Intentions and Desires are supported
> [Om Rih-tam Na-ma-ha]   by the Universe."

6. Friday – The Law of Detachment

The Law of Detachment is the Principle of Freedom. Learn that you don't have to be rigidly attached to how you are "supposed to be." Feel the power in allowing yourself and all others to be who they are. Notice what lights you up and follow that light. Find what feels natural for you. There is a lot of power in the words "I am free to be me." Commit to detachment and embrace uncertainty; it is essential to your path to freedom. Do not force situations; allow them to spontaneously emerge. Step into the field of all possibilities. Know that when things don't seem to go your way, something much better is awaiting you. Your life will be full of adventure, magic, and mystery.

1) Commit yourself to detachment. 2) Factor in and accept uncertainty.
3) Remain open to all possibilities.

> **MANTRA:**
> Om Anandham Namaha   "My actions are blissfully free from.
> [Om Ah-nan-dam Na-ma-ha]   from attachment to outcome."

7. Saturday – The Law of Dharma or Purpose in Life

You are here to fulfill a purpose; you hold a unique talent with a unique expression. To find your dharma you can create a list of everything you love and enjoy doing. Then ask yourself: "If I can do anything in the world and money is no object – what would that be?" Combine your answer with the list of the things you love to do. Then ask… "How can I help? How can I serve?" Begin to understand and honor your unique way of performing the job you are in. You may then realize how important your part is that you are performing. Honor your uniqueness and realize your importance. Discover your Higher Self and express your unique talents.

1) Notice what lights you up. 2) Honor your unique expression.

3) Ask "How can I help? How can I serve?"

MANTRA:

Om Varunam Namaha   "My life is in harmony with the Universe."
[Om Var-u-nam Na-ma-ha]

Read one principle per day and incorporate the 3 applications into your daily life. The Laws will take on new meaning… similar to how each day has new meaning as you grow, evolve, and transform. Enjoy the beautiful journey.

"We have stopped for a moment to encounter each other, to meet, to love, to share.
This is a precious moment. It is a little parenthesis in eternity.
If we share with caring, lightheartedness and love, we will create abundance
and joy for each other. And then this moment will have been worthwhile."

-Dr. Deepak Chopra, *The Seven Spiritual Laws of Success*

DAILY ROUTINE

1. Drink 8 ounces of Room Temperature Water in the Morning.

2. 5-10 Minutes of Breathing Techniques.

3. 10-20 Minutes of Meditation / Gratitude.

4. 10-15 Minutes of Movement; 6 Directions of the Spine.

5. 2-6 Sun Salutations.

6. Stay Present Throughout the Day.

7. Drink 1 to 2 Glasses of Water Between Meals.

8. Eat Whole Foods and Give Thanks Before Eating.

9. Keep One Principle from *"The Seven Spiritual Laws of Success" (Deepak Chopra)* in Your Awareness.

10. Meditate in the Evening, Before or After Dinner.

11. Before Bed, Feel Gratitude for All That You Have.

12. Take a Warm Bath or Shower Before Bed.

"Walk and touch peace in every moment. Walk and touch Happiness in every moment. Each step brings a fresh breeze. Each step makes a flower bloom under our feet."

-Thich Nhat Han